STRETCH MARKS REMOVAL

How to remove your stretch marks fast

Monica Evans

For Notes

Copyright ® 2019

DISCLAIMER

The information that this Book contained is strictly for remedy purposes for stretch marks removalThe author has wholly made every effort to safeguard the accuracy of the information within this book at the time of publication has used research information.

The author does not assume and at this moment disclaims any form of the liabilities to any either party for any damage, loss, or disruption caused by omissions or errors, whether the mistakes or omissions occurred from misconstruing, or any other causes.

CONTENTS

INTRODUCTION

An introduction to the removal of the Stretch mark

People are looking for a stretch mark removal cream that works since we were graced with beauty by Aphrodite and Cleopatra. Stretch marks are lines that form on the surface of the skin in a nutshell. They are usually caused by stretching your skin due to several reasons.

The Skin Structure, it is important to understand the layers of the skin and the role they play in our body to better understand why they can develop. The skin consists of three major layers:

• An outer layer called the epidermis that helps protect your body;

• An inner layer of fat and connecting tissues ("hypodermis")

• The dermis, the middle layer of skin that supports and gives flexibility to the structure

The middle layer called "dermis" is the skin layer that affects d by stretch marks. You may notice violet or red lines appearing as stretch marks as parts of your middle layer breaks. This coloring is due to your blood vessels that may eventually contract and may turn white on your stretch marks.

What are the causes?

Stretch marks occur down to the skin breaking dermis layer. History of the family and choices of lifestyle are some of the reasons for this. They are common throughout the world and are not limited to women alone. On the thighs, buttocks and tummy, the more common areas they appear. Pregnant mothers will usually experience them as their skin expands to accommodate their babies. They may also develop them as further hormonal activity makes their skin more prone to stretching.

Weight gain is also a significant reason to develop them, especially if the weight gain occurs in a concise time. People who diet continuously may experience stretch marks as their weight fluctuates and may also result from the rapid growth of the muscle. During puberty, many people will notice stretch marks as they overgrow during their lifetime. They may also occur due to family genetics and some medication and may even be a sign of the syndrome of a person with Cushing. In this specific instance, the body will produce too many hormones.

There are several causes, as you have seen, and they're just a fact of life for many. They will slowly fade for most people, while some might feel a lack of trust due to stretch marks throughout their body. There are also a lot of options available for the removal of stretch marks, such as lotions, cosmetic surgery, laser therapy, and perhaps more.

Fortunately, stretch marks can be treated as well. There is nothing to fear about the stretch marks. By choosing safe stretch mark removal with natural remedies, you can prevent or eliminate the effects of stretch marks.

Given below are the active home remedies for stretch marks removal for women

Baby Oil
Cocoa Butter
Turmeric

Tea Tree Oil

Castor Oil

Aloe Vera

Coffee Scrub

Almond Oil

Vicks Vaporub

Vitamin E Oil

Baking Soda

Glycolic Acid

Apple Cider Vinegar

Jojoba Oil

Rosehip Oil

Olive Oil

Juice

Argan Oil

Shea Butter

Apricot Mask and Oil

Cucumber and Lemon Sugar Scrub

Lemon

COCOA BUTTER FOR STRETCH MARKS

INGREDIENTS:

1/2 cup cocoa butter

1 tablespoon apricot oil

1 tablespoon wheat germ oil

1 tablespoon kernel oil

1 tablespoon vitamin E oil

2 teaspoons beeswax

PREPARATION

Prepare a mixture of the ingredients and heat it till the wax has liquefied totally.

Store the mixture in an airtight container in your refrigerator. Rub on the mixture on the stretch marks and massage for a few minutes till the skin well absorbs it.

How Frequently You Need to Do This

Apply this twice or thrice a day.

Reason this works

For the stretch marks, Cocoa butter is also extremely active. Your skin will be hydrated and made smoother. It penetrates the deeper layers of the skin and replenishes and repairs damaged cells.

SHEA BUTTER FOR STRETCH MARKS

INGREDIENTS

Shea butter

PREPARATION

Massage or apply Shea butter on the affected areas properly and leave it on the skin.

How Frequently You Need to Do This

Reapply a few times during the day.

Why this is working

Shea butter includes antioxidant and anti-inflammatory properties in addition to being highly moisturizing for the skin. The consistent application will keep your skin healthy and repair any damaged cells.

ALOE VERA FOR STRETCH MARKS

INGREDIENTS

Fresh aloe vera gel

5 vitamins A capsules

10 vitamin E capsules

PREPARATION

Take out the new gel from an aloe vera leaf and, add to it oil from vitamin A and E capsules. Mix it well. Massage this on the affected skin until the mixture is completely absorbed. You shouldn't rinse it. You can apply aloe vera gel as well. Leave it on and wash with warm water for 15 minutes.

How Frequently You Need to Do This.

Repeat this twice a day until the stretch marks start fading away and vanish.

Why this works

Aloe Vera gel is a very beneficial herb for the body, especially the skin. It is soothing to the surface, and the healing process is also applied. This is due to the influence of substances of glucomannan and gibberellin that boost collagen synthesis and stretch marks of fade. It also includes essential vitamins, minerals, and antioxidant enzymes.

CASTOR OIL FOR STRETCH MARKS

INGREDIENTS

Castor oil

PREPARATION

Heat the castor oil slightly and massage it with the stretch marks. Leave it for about 15 minutes to 20 minutes.

How Frequently You Need to Do This

Doing this guide every day before going to bed to make work better.

Reason this works

Castor oil is frequently used to treat skin diseases and hair fall. It also contains ricinoleic acid, a skin-conditioning agent that fastens the healing of stretch marks and makes them appear a lot lighter.

COFFEE SCRUB FOR STRETCH MARKS

INGREDIENTS

Coffee grounds

Water

PREPARATION

Make a paste by mixing coffee with water. Massage this well over the affected area. Massage in gentle, rub in a circular motion between three to five minutes.

Thoroughly rinse and moisturize with actual warm water. For better results, you can add one or two tablespoons of olive oil or aloe vera gel.

How Frequently You Need to Do This

Use this scrub every day.

Reason this works

Coffee is very rich in caffeine which has high biological activity and can penetrate the skin quickly. It arouses the degradation of fats under the skin and also has antioxidant properties. The gentle massaging motion will also enhance the blood flow in that area. All of these lighten the stretch marks.

SUGAR SCRUB FOR STRETCH MARKS

INGREDIENTS

1 tablespoon raw sugar

A few drops of almond oil

A few drops of lemon juice

PREPARATION

Mix all the ingredients to make a grainy scrub. Massage this into your skin for 8-10 minutes. Wash with tepid water and moisturize as usual.

How many times you can go on this?

Practice this scrub at once or twice a day.

Reason this works

Sugar acts as an excellent exfoliant and helps in the shedding of dead cells. It improves circulation and boosts the healing capacity of the stretch marks.

TEA TREE OIL FOR STRETCH MARKS

INGREDIENTS

4-5 drops of tea tree oil

1 ½ tablespoons olive oil or coconut oil

PREPARATION

Mix the carrier oil with essential oil and rub stretch marks. Let the skin take it up and let it get on.

How often You can Perform This

Apply this 2 times a day.

Why this works

Tea tree oil has several benefits. Its potential to disappear stretch marks and scars is one of the better-known benefits. It also includes anti-inflammatory properties.

ARGAN OIL FOR STRETCH MARKS

INGREDIENTS

Organic Argan oil

PREPARATION

Apply the oil to the stretch marks and massage for 60 seconds. The oil gets quickly absorbed into the skin. Do not wipe away or rinse.

How Frequently You Need to Do This

Do this twice daily to get rid of stretch marks.

Reason this works

Argan oil is commonly used in cosmetic products for its benefits. It is rich in vitamin E and has antioxidant properties. This will nourish and heal the skin and decrease scars and stretch marks at the same time. The collagen and elastic fibers

of the surface are re-energized by Argan
Oil application.

VICKS VAPORUB FOR STRETCH MARKS

INGREDIENTS

Vicks Vaporub

Cling wrap

PREPARATION

Apply the vaporub on the stretch mark and rub in for two minutes. Use cling wrap to cover the area and leave it overnight.

How Frequently You Need to Do This

Repeat this guide every night till the stretch marks fade away.

Reason this works

Vicks Vaporub contains essential oils namely eucalyptus oil, turpentine oil, and cedar leaf oil. It has camphor and petrolatum. All these works together to moisturize the skin and makes it softer.

Although no scientific data are available to support this remedy, women around the world have noticed a 60-80 percent difference in their stretch marks by using this medication.

VITAMIN E OIL FOR STRETCH MARKS

INGREDIENTS

Vitamin E oil capsules

PREPARATION

Cut the capsule to extract the oil. Apply this oil to your stretch marks and rub in for some minutes. Let it be on. You can consider taking a capsule of vitamin E oil every day.

How Frequently You Need to Do This

Apply this oil twice or thrice daily.

Why does that work?

Vitamin E oil is typically found in creams and lotions for removing scratches and preventing skin ageing. It has anti-inflammatory and antimicrobial properties that feed the skin, keep it healthy, and help with scars and stretch marks recovery process.

OLIVE OIL FOR STRETCH MARKS

INGREDIENTS

Extra virgin olive oil

PREPARATION

Let the oil be lightly warm and rub it on the affected area for a few minutes. Do not wash it off.

How Regularly You Need To Do This

Repeat this twice a day.

The reason this does effectively

Olive oil is nutrient-rich, vitamin-rich, and antioxidant. For the skin, it is very healthy and helps to relieve several skin problems such as stretch marks. It has anti inflammatory properties.

ALMOND OIL FOR STRETCH MARKS

INGREDIENTS

1-2 tablespoons sweet almond oil

A few drops of essential oil

PREPARATION

Sweet almond oil, mix a few drops of your favorite essential oil and stir well. Put on the cooker for a few seconds and apply all over the stretch marks. Massage in a circular motion for some minutes and wait till it dry.

How Frequently You Need to Do This

Do this twice per day.

Reason this works

This has been verified to lessen scarring and to improve and care for the complexion of the skin. Almond oil comprises Vitamin E and essential nutrients that nourish and rebuild the surface quickly.

BABY OIL FOR STRETCH MARKS

INGREDIENTS

Baby oil

PREPARATION

Shower with hot water, after that, pat your skin dry and apply baby oil to the affected area. Massage thoroughly so that the oil gets absorbed into the skin. Leave the oil to dry naturally.

How Frequently You Need to Do This

Use the oil daily after taking a shower.

Reason this works

The baby oil contains essential nutrients that will nourish your skin and keep it soft and agile. It will deter the appearance of stretch marks.

BAKING SODA FOR STRETCH MARKS

INGREDIENTS

Juice of one lemon

1 tablespoon baking soda

Cling wrap

PREPARATION

Combine baking soda with lemon juice, then stir to form a paste. Apply this on the affected spot, wrap in cling, and let it stay for 20-30 minutes in the area. Remove the wrap and warm water for rinsing.

How Frequently You Need to Do This

You need to apply this regularly for quick removal of stretch marks on you.

The reason it is efficient

Baking soda by exfoliating the skin will remove the dead skin layer, therefore, lightening the stretch marks of the body.

GLYCOLIC ACID FOR STRETCH MARKS

INGREDIENTS

Glycolic acid

PREPARATION

You are to apply the liquid to the affected area and leave it to dry.

How Frequently You Need To Do This

You have to repeat this process every day, preferably before going to bed.

Reason this works

This chemical is readily available in a medical store and is considered safe to apply, even during pregnancy. It intensifies the collagen in your skin, making it more elastic and healthier.

Warning

Protect your skin with the right gear if you cannot avoid stepping out in the sunlight. After applying this do not go out in the sun as it can easily cause sunburns.

LEMON ON STRETCH MARKS

INGREDIENTS

1-2 tablespoons fresh lemon juice

PREPARATION

Smear the lemon juice in circular motions on the stretch marks. Let the skin grip it for about 10 minutes. Rinse with warm water. Apply a moisturizer. Add a teaspoon of cucumber juice and then add one or two teaspoons of gram flour to this and make a paste. Apply this to your skin, let it dry for 10 minutes, and rinse with warm water.

How often You should go on

Repeat this twice per day.

Reason this works

Lemon juice is naturally acidic, which helps to heal and diminish stretch marks, acne, and other scars.

APPLE CIDER VINEGAR FOR STRETCH

MARKS

INGREDIENTS

1 cup apple cider vinegar

A spray bottles

PREPARATION

Into the spray bottle, add the apple cider vinegar. Sprinkle over your stretch marks and let it dry on its own. Shower thoroughly in the morning and moisturize the skin.

How Frequently you need this

Do this before going to bed every night.

The reason that makes this to work is that ACV is rich in acetic and malic acid, which helps remove the scars.

TURMERIC FOR STRETCH MARKS

INGREDIENTS

Ground Turmeric

PREPARATION

Wash with warm water and moisturize.

How Frequently You Need to Do This

Repeat this two times daily to get rid of the stretch marks.

Reason this works

Turmeric is comprised of antioxidants and also contain anti-inflammatory and skin-lightening properties. Regular application of turmeric makes the best way to get rid of stretch marks. After a few weeks, you will even notice your stretch marks has faded away to a great extent.

JOJOBA OIL FOR STRETCH MARKS

INGREDIENTS

Pure jojoba oil

PREPARATION

Take some drops of the oil and rub it on the stretch marks. Massage for some minutes and leave it on.

How Frequently

Rub on the oil two to three times every day.

Reason

Jojoba oil has anti-inflammatory and skin cure properties. It is strongly encouraged that when the stretch marks start appearing, you start rubbing on this. It will nourish and heal your skin and boost the growth of healthier new cells. This will also prevent them from spreading further.

ROSEHIP OIL FOR STRETCH MARKS

INGREDIENTS

Rosehip oil

PREPARATION

Apply a few drops of this rosehip oil on the stretch marks in a circular, massaging motion. Rub in and leave it on your skin to dry.

How Frequently You Need to Do This

Apply this twice per day.

Reason this is very active

Rosehip oil provides antioxidants, vitamins A and E to your skin, which boosts collagen production. It increases the skin's healing capacity and reduces stretch marks and other scars.

CUCUMBER AND LEMON JUICE

INGREDIENTS

Lemon juice

Cucumber Juice

PREPARATION

Mix cucumber juice with lime juice in equal parts, and rub the mixture on the affected areas of your skin till it gets absorbed by the skin. Let it be on your skin for 10 minutes after which you can rinse it off with tepid water.

How Frequently You Need to Do This

To get good results, repeat the procedure every day for at least a month.

Reason this is effective

Lemon juice's natural acidity helps to heal and reduce scars and cucumber juice. It provides a cooling, soothing effect leaving your skin fresh.

APRICOT MASK AND OIL

INGREDIENTS

Apricots mask

Oil

PREPARATION

Cut 2-3 apricots, then take out the seeds. Crush the fruit into a paste. Mix the glue and oil in equal parts, then apply this mask to the areas affected with stretch marks and leave it for 15 minutes. Using tepid water, rinse it off.

How Frequently You Need to Do This

Perform the process every day for a month for good results.

Why this works

Pure Apricot oil rejuvenates the skin and helps to reduce stretch marks. Apricots have great tendencies to exfoliate, making them very effective in healing stretch marks. You can also apply some lemon juice to the skin for effective results.

NOURISHING SKIN MASK

INGREDIENTS

2tsp oatmeal

2tsp almond paste

Juice of one lemon

2 egg yolks, beaten

Add enough milk and mix to a smooth paste

PREPARATION

Put together all the ingredients and mix well. Apply on the stretch marks. Allow it to dry completely. Wash with cold water while scrubbing gently.

How Frequently You Need to apply it?

You should do this on alternate days.

ALMOND OIL WITH ALOE VERA GEL

INGREDIENTS

Aloe Vera gel. 1tsp

Almond oil 1 tsp

PROCEDURE

Inside a clean bowl: add 1 tsp of aloe vera gel, and 1 tsp of almond oil. Mix very well, until it smoothens. Apply this mixture to your skin daily,

How Frequently You Need to Do This

Repeat the process every day.

POTATO JUICE

INGREDIENTS

Potato

PROCEDURE

Peel off the potato covering. Cut into small pieces. With a blender jar, put the potato pieces in it and blend well, make juice of it. Rub the juice on the stretch marks and allow it to dry. After that, rinse off with cold water.

How Frequently You Need to Do This

Repeat the process.

Why These Works.

It contains a high content of vitamins and minerals like calcium, potassium, phosphorus, magnesium.

EGG WHITE

INGREDIENTS

Egg white

PREPARATION

Take an egg, remove the white separately in a bowl, whisk together then apply the mixture to the affected area. Let it dry for 15-25 minutes. Take a shower after that.

How Frequently You Need to Do This

Repeat the process each day for a month.

Why it is effective

It has 40 proteins, Amino Acids, Vitamin A, and Collagen. These are the best way to get rid of stretch marks instantly.

SUGAR AND LEMON JUICE

INGREDIENTS

1. Sugar

2. Lemon juice

3. Almond oil

PREPARATION

Add some lemon juice to some sugar in a bowl, mix well till the sugar is wholly dissolved in the lemon juice.

Add small drops of almond oil, and mix well, then apply this mixture to the affected skin. Leave it for some minutes, and wash off with tepid water.

How Frequently You Need to Do This

Repeat this daily to remove the stretch marks.

GALLIC PASTE

INGREDIENTS

1. Garlic 20 cloves

PREPARATION

Make a paste of garlic using a mixer.

Apply it to the stretch marks and wash after 30 minutes.

How Frequently You Need to Do This

Repeat the process daily for good results.

COFFEE GROUNDS WITH WARM WATER

INGREDIENTS

1. Coffee

2. Warm water.

PREPARATION

Mix coffee grounds with warm water in a bowl, then drink the coffee. It lessens the stretch marks.

How Frequently You Need to Do This

Repeat this guide every day for a good result.

COFFEE GROUNDS AND ALOE VERA GEL

INGREDIENTS

1. Coffee grounds

2. Aloe Vera Gel

PREPARATION

Take a bowl, put some coffee ground in it, and aloe vera gel in the same amount. Mix with aloe vera gel, and make a paste that will help you massage the coffee grounds onto your stretch marks.

Apply the coffee, and Aloe Vera paste to your skin. Shower first and pat your body dry before applying the mixture. Use your fingers to spread the coffee and Aloe Vera mixture based unto your stretch marks.

Then allow the mixture to remain on your skin for 20 minutes. You can then wipe off with a clean cloth moistened with water.

How Frequently You Need to Do This

You are to do this once per day. After that, you need to apply this moist skin lotion once or twice per day.

The Reason Why This works

Aloe Vera contains Vitamin C and E. It moisturizes the skin.

MOISTURES

INGREDIENTS

1. Avocado oil. 1 tsp

2. Cocoa butter. 1 cup

3. Aloe Vera gel. 1 tsp

4. Vitamin E. 3 capsules

5. Lavender and tea tree 1 tsp

6. Pure Shea butter. 1 cup

7. Organic coconut oil. 1 cup

PREPARATION

Put all ingredients in a pot, then bring to steam and stir all the ingredients together till everything is liquefied, pour into a container, and put it in a refrigerator to freeze. Then, apply it on the stretch mark infected area, leave and let it dry totally.

How Frequently You Need to Apply This

You can do this almost all the time.

Why These Works

This Coconut Oil helps in moisturizing, healing, and providing cool, soothing effect of leaving your skin fresh.

Cocoa Butter and Lavender Oil helps avoid and lessen the presence of scars and stretch marks. Aloe Vera Gel is good for rejuvenation of skin tissues. Shea Butter substitutes missing fatty acids in the skin, while Avocado Oil improves the elasticity of the skin, and Vitamin E is a powerful antioxidant.

All these make them very active when it comes to healing stretch marks.

RAW SUGAR & SHEA BUTTER

INGREDIENTS

1/4 cup olive oil or coconut oil

1/2 teaspoon vitamin E oil

1/2 cup organic raw cane sugar

5 drops lavender essential oil

1 teaspoon organic lemon juice or 3 drops of lemon essential oil

1 tablespoon shea butter

PREPARATION

Add ingredients in a bowl and mix very well. For better results, place in a pan at low heat, stirring until smooth. Put all ingredients in a glass jar or container with a lid.

Rub on affected areas two to three times per week.

SUGAR AND HONEY

INGREDIENTS

Sugar

Honey

PREPARATION

In a small bowl, add 1 table cubit honey to 1 table cubit sugar. Remove it well. To make a thinner consistency glue, add 1 tablespoon of olive oil or coconut oil

Apply the mixture and the affected area of the stretch mark and massage for 5 minutes in a circular motion. Leave it for another five minutes.

Why These Works

Honey helps to retain moisture assisting the sagged skin in tightening. Do it every other day

OLIVE OIL PLUS SUGAR

INGREDIENTS

Olive Oil

Sugar

PREPARATION

In a minor bowl, add one tablespoon of olive oil to 1 tablespoon of sugar. To make a thin paste, stir well. Rub it 10 minutes on the affected stretch mark area. Leave it there for like 5 minutes, and rinse it off with water. Adding olive oil is intended to attract moisture in one area to concentrate.

Why These Works

Moisture helps to reconstruct skin cells more quickly. Do it every day.

SUGAR AND CASTOR OIL

INGREDIENTS

Sugar

Castor Oil

PREPARATION

Mix castor oil tablespoon with 1 tablespoon of fine granulated sugar. Apply the assortment on the stretch marks and massage in a circular motion for 5 minutes. Wash it off with water. The skin is moisturized by castor oil.

Why These Works

The castor oil's ricinoleic acid penetrates the skin to tightness it and decreases stretch marks. Apply it daily.

SUGAR AND COCONUT OIL

INGREDIENTS

Sugar

Coconut oil

PREPARATION

Mix one tablespoon of coconut oil and 1 tablespoon of sugar well. Cover the bowl and keep the mixture for 60 seconds for sugar and coconut oil to blend well. Stir well again before use because some sugar may have settled down at the bottom of the bowl.

Massage it in the affected area for 10 minutes.

Rinse if with water after 5 minutes. Coconut oil is very active in enlightening elasticity in the skin due to monosaturated fats.

SUGAR AND ALMOND OIL

INGREDIENTS

Sugar

Almond oil

PREPARATION

In equal quantities, add fine granulated sugar and almond oil. To make a thick paste, mix well. Massage 5 minutes with the paste of the affected stretch marked area. After 5 minutes, wash with water. Do it 2-3 times per week.

Why These Works

An excellent skin repair oil is the nutritious almond oil. Giving skin its smoothness and glow are rich in vitamin A and E.

CONCLUSION

These are the best home remedies to get clear of stretch marks. Put them into your daily routine to prevent stretch marks from appearing and also vanishing of any marks that had appeared already.

Natural treatments for stretch marks are an excellent home remedy. As a result of the skin stretching to accommodate changes in our body, these unsightly lines often appear on our thighs, hips, stomach, breasts, arms, and/or buttocks. Pregnancy, weight gain, and even body building muscle growth or weight training can lead to stretch marks.

However, like other scars, you can help them to disappear or at least lighten up so that some home treatments don't make them as noticeable. As a law, you want to find as soon as possible a stretch mark cure. So, treat them as soon as you notice them and you can deal more effectively with them.